COMPLETE DIABETES MANAGEMENT

BLOOD SUGAR REGULATION AND STABILIZATION

By

Anthony M. Smith

TABLE OF CONTENT

INTRODUCTION

Diabetes one of the fastest-growing diseases overall is expanding swiftly in people of all age bunches including adolescents and kids. The issue develops when the body does not supply adequate insulin or cannot use it properly. From heart infection, renal difficulties, and stroke to bringing down appendage removal, the persistent illness provides many well-being risks to persons affected by it.

This book contains instructions about how to manage diabetes. However, this is not the case. Many individuals have lived long healthy lives even after being diagnosed with diabetes by just modifying their lifestyle. This certainly does not imply that adopting a new lifestyle is a piece of cake. It is obviously tough but what other alternative do you have? Continue living an unhealthy life and die only a few years down the line?

COMPLETE DIABETES MANAGEMENT will help you learn more about diabetes, some wonderful eating, exercising, and general suggestions to help you manage and control your diabetes so that you may have a normally long and satisfying life. Thank you for getting this book, I hope you like it.

DIABETES

Everyone's heard of diabetes. It's one of the most prevalent chronic illnesses in the world and rates are continuing on the increase. Yet most individuals don't completely comprehend what causes it or how it impacts ordinary life. Many assume that since the condition is so common, it isn't severe. But if left untreated, diabetes may lead to heart problems, eyesight loss, and even limb amputation.

At its most basic, diabetes mellitus (the official term) is a series of illnesses that cause individuals to have higher-than-normal quantities of sugar—or, glucose—in their blood. Glucose originates from the protein, carbs, and fats that you consume and drink, as well as your liver, which creates and stores the material.

If everything is going according to plan, your pancreas produces a hormone called insulin that helps transfer glucose from the circulation into certain of the cells of your body to be utilized for energy. But if your body is resistant to insulin, or doesn't create enough of it, the glucose is trapped hanging around in your blood. That's when your doctor will inform you that you have "high blood sugar." As time goes on, the additional sugar in your blood creates inflammation and other severe health concerns.

About 30 million individuals in the United States have diabetes, yet roughly one-quarter of them don't know it. Let's take a deeper look.

Types of Diabetes

There are various distinct varieties of diabetes and each has its own causes. It's vital to acquire a precise diagnosis for the kind of illness you have since treatment may change based on type. Here are the essentials you should know:

PREDIABETES

If someone's blood sugar is higher than usual, but not high enough to be classified as type 2 diabetes, that's termed prediabetes. That indicates an A1C blood test result between 5.7% and 6.4%. More than one in three persons in the United States has prediabetes, and the majority of them don't know it, That's a concern since people with prediabetes have an increased chance of developing type 2. Luckily, prediabetes may be reversed: Exercise and diet adjustments are typically suggested to decrease blood sugar and lessen the risk. In rare circumstances, a doctor may additionally prescribe metformin, a blood-sugar-lowering medicine to help prevent type 2.

You're at risk of prediabetes if you:

having mother, father or siblings with type 2 diabetes

Have ever had gestational diabetes

Are 45 or older

Are overweight

Aren't physically active at least three times each week

TYPE 1 DIABETES

Also called "juvenile" diabetes because it's commonly diagnosed in infancy, type 1 diabetes is largely an autoimmune illness in which your immune system targets and kills insulin-making cells in the pancreas. Because of this, your body no longer manufactures its own insulin, thus you require insulin injections every day. It's assumed that a mix of genetics and environmental factors may cause the condition to develop in the first place.

Most persons with type 1 diabetes are diagnosed during childhood or early adulthood, however, a small proportion of people may not acquire the condition until their 30s, 40s, or even 50s.

TYPE 1 DIABETES COMPLICATIONS

Having type 1 diabetes also puts you at risk for various health complications, particularly if left untreated. Some probable problems include:

- **Cardiovascular disease:** People with diabetes are at higher risk of heart disease, stroke, and high blood pressure.
- **Diabetic neuropathy:** Over time, having high blood sugar may lead to nerve damage, termed diabetic neuropathy. This shows sensations of tingling, discomfort, numbness, or burning and affects around one-half of patients with diabetes. Additionally, nerve damage that happens in the feet may lead to inadequate blood flow which can result in a higher risk of foot issues such as serious

infections from wounds and
blisters.

- **Kidney disease
  (nephropathy):** Having diabetes
  increases you more prone to
  develop chronic kidney disease.
  That's because diabetes may harm
  the filtration mechanism in your
  kidneys that eliminates waste from
  your blood.

- **Eye difficulties:** Your eyes are
  also at higher risk of health
  problems with diabetes, such as
  glaucoma and cataracts. You also
  may encounter damage to the
  blood vessels in the portion of
  your eye called the retina, a
  disease known as diabetic
  retinopathy, which may result in
  loss of sight.

- **Skin problems:** People with diabetes are more prone to skin infections and other illnesses.
- **Pregnancy complications:** Type 1 diabetes may lead to concerns for you and your baby if you are pregnant. For example, your risk of miscarriage, stillbirth, and birth abnormalities is increased if your diabetes is uncontrolled during pregnancy.

TYPE 2 DIABETES

It's rare to claim there's "good news" about any medical diagnosis, but if there's a silver lining with type 2 diabetes, it's this: You are very much in charge of your fate. Type 2 diabetes may frequently be effectively

treated by the activities you take in daily life. A good diet and regular exercise, together with prescribed drugs, may give you your life back.

If you know someone with diabetes, probability they have type 2, which accounts for 90% to 95% of all diabetes cases in the United States. Other prevalent forms include type 1, an autoimmune condition, and gestational diabetes, which only arises during pregnancy.

People with all forms of diabetes have one thing in common: excessive quantities of sugar (or glucose) in the blood.

Here's what occurs if your body is operating normally: After you eat, food from your meal is broken down into a sugar called glucose (among other things) that serves as your whole body's source of energy—the brain, heart, muscle cells, and everything else relies on glucose for fuel.

The glucose enters the circulation and in reaction, your pancreas produces insulin, a hormone that helps the glucose move out of your blood and into certain cells so they can utilize it for energy.

But with type 2 diabetes, your body quits utilizing the insulin it creates effectively, needing more and more insulin to help convert glucose into energy. Eventually, your pancreas can't create enough insulin to keep up with the demand, and your blood sugar increases. (This is different from type 1, when the body doesn't create insulin at all, leading glucose to build up in the blood.)

Type 2 diabetes is relatively manageable, but not curable. Some individuals are able to keep it in control with a balanced diet and frequent exercise, but many need to take medication as well.

It's vital to be identified early and accurately because, if left untreated, type 2 diabetes dramatically raises your risk of heart disease and may lead to consequences including eyesight loss, kidney troubles, nerve pain, foot problems, and even amputations.

TYPE 2 DIABETES COMPLICATIONS

It's crucial to manage type 2 diabetes because, like type 1, it may wreak havoc on your body in numerous ways. People with type 2 diabetes have the same long-term effects of diabetes as type 1 (see above list), including diabetic neuropathy, skin issues, renal disease, eye difficulties, cardiovascular disease, and more.

GESTATIONAL DIABETES

Gestational diabetes refers to transitory elevated blood sugar that arises exclusively in pregnancy. Doctors assume that it's connected to hormonal changes that occur during this period. Every year, around 2% to 10% of pregnant women in the United States may have gestational diabetes.

Most pregnant women are evaluated for gestational diabetes during their second trimester with a glucose tolerance test, which includes drinking a glucose-containing beverage on an empty stomach and then having blood collected to examine sugar levels.

Gestational diabetes is commonly managed with exercise and nutrition adjustments (such as consuming fewer carbs and more vegetables, fruits, and protein). Some women may require insulin shots, too.

Most of the time, blood sugar levels return to normal after the baby is delivered; however, if you have gestational diabetes during pregnancy, you are also at higher-than-average risk for acquiring type 2 later in life. In fact, roughly 50% of patients with gestational diabetes end up developing type 2.

Gestational diabetes also puts your baby at risk of health complications. For example, infant with mothers who have gestational diabetes have a higher probability of low blood sugar, preterm birth (which can lead to breathing trouble and other issues), being delivered more than nine pounds (which can lead to hard delivery or C-section), and getting type 2 diabetes in future.

Other Types of Diabetes

Though uncommon, these kinds of diabetes may cause major health complications if left untreated:

• **Monogenic diabetes:** Accounting for 1% to 5% of all cases, this unusual kind of diabetes is caused by a mutation in a single gene. In most situations, the illness is related to a person's pancreas not being able to create enough insulin; the ailment is commonly observed in youngsters. If untreated, monogenic diabetes may lead to damage to the blood vessels in your eyes and kidneys.

• **Secondary diabetes:** Sometimes, diabetes is a side-effect of another condition, such as Cushing's syndrome and cystic fibrosis. These kinds of diabetes have a comparable risk of complications as other forms of diabetes.

• **Cystic fibrosis-related diabetes:** If you have cystic fibrosis, you are at risk of this kind of diabetes. Basically, the scarring of the pancreas that happens in cystic fibrosis might make it challenging for your pancreas to create the insulin you require. Cystic fibrosis-related diabetes exhibits certain hallmarks of type 1 diabetes and other signs of type 2 diabetes.

CAUSES OF DIABETES

The causes of diabetes range depending on what kind you have. No matter what kind it is, however, difficulties with insulin constitute the basis of the condition. With type 1 diabetes, it's thought that a mix of environmental stimuli (such as viruses) and your genes cause the body to start attacking insulin-producing cells. With type 2, lifestyle factors and heredity contribute to insulin issues. Typically, this begins with insulin resistance, in which your body simply doesn't utilize insulin as effectively as it should.

Causes of Type 1 diabetes

Type 1 diabetes is largely an autoimmune condition. In this situation, your immune system assaults your body in the same way it may target intruders like germs or viruses, killing specific cells in your pancreas in a mistaken effort to defend the body. These cells, termed beta cells, are the ones that create insulin. When your body attacks and kills them, you can no longer create your own insulin.

Doctors think that type 1 diabetes may be caused by a mix of genetic and environmental factors. Type 1 diabetes is controllable with daily insulin injections but isn't curable, and lifestyle modifications like diet and exercise won't cure it.

Causes of Type 2 diabetes

Type 2 diabetes is frequently caused by a combination of causes. It tends to run in families, and certain genes make you more prone to get it. It's also more frequent in several ethnic groups, including Native Americans, African Americans, Pacific Islanders, Asians, and Latinos.

How you eat and how active you are also crucial. Carrying additional body fat, particularly in your belly, may lead to insulin resistance, a scenario where your pancreas creates enough insulin, but doesn't utilize it efficiently, so sugar builds up in your blood rather than moving into your cells for energy. Insulin resistance is a main factor of type 2 diabetes.

Sometimes, type 2 diabetes is caused by an underactive pancreas and your body doesn't create enough insulin.

• **Ethnicity/race.** Certain ethnic groups are more prone to acquire type 2 than others, including African Americans, Latinos, Pacific Islanders and Hawaiians, Native Americans, and Native Alaskans.

• **Family history and genetics**. There is no one type 2 diabetes "gene" to test for, but if type 2 runs in your family, that indicates you are at increased risk of having it, too.

• **High Body Mass Index (BMI).** Higher amounts of body fat, particularly the sort that collects in the belly, are associated with insulin resistance and risk of type 2 diabetes. Insulin resistance may also induce greater weight gain, creating a vicious cycle.

• **Insulin resistance**. Type 2 frequently begins with insulin resistance—meaning that a person's liver, muscles, adipose (fat), and other cells start to react more slowly or weakly to insulin than they used to. Several causes may lead to insulin resistance, including some drugs, polycystic ovarian syndrome, Cushing's disease, and age.

• **Sedentary lifestyle**. Physical exercise enhances your body's capacity to utilize insulin effectively, decreasing the risk of high blood sugar. Being inactive makes your cells less responsive to insulin, which leads to insulin resistance and higher risk of type 2 diabetes.

Causes of Gestational Diabetes

Genetics and hormonal changes during pregnancy are the causes of this kind. You're at higher risk of having this kind of diabetes if you

• Have had it in a former pregnancy

• If you are overweight earlier pregnancy

• Have polycystic ovary syndrome

• Have given birth to a kids over nine pounds

• Have a family report of type 2
diabetes

All women become insulin-resistant late
in pregnancy, due to hormones secreted
largely by the placenta. Most of the
time, the pancreas amps up the
production of insulin to make up the
difference, but in cases where it can't
keep up, blood sugar levels rise and
gestational diabetes develops.

RISK FACTORS

Now that we know what causes diabetes
to develop in the first place, you're
certainly wondering if you are at risk of
acquiring this particular ailment. It's true
that there are several circumstances
that might make you more prone to
have diabetes. Knowing your risk factors
empowers you with knowledge—
knowledge you can use to take

measures to lower that risk and be as healthy as possible. Here's what you need to know.

Type 1 Diabetes Risk Factors

Compared with type 2 diabetes, risk factors for type 1 diabetes are a little less understood. That so, a handful of the primary risk factors are clear:

• **Family history:** If your parent or sibling has type 1 diabetes, you're also more likely to have the illness.

• **Younger age**: Children, teenagers, and young adults are the most likely to have type 1 diabetes (that's why it's frequently called "juvenile diabetes"), but it's possible to get it at any age.

• **Race**: In the United States, you're more likely to have type 1 if you are white compared with Black and Latinx Americans.

Type 2 Diabetes Risk Factors

Risk factors for acquiring type 2 diabetes include: • Prediabetes. Having prediabetes dramatically enhances your risk of going on to develop full-blown type 2.

• **Being overweight**: Having extra weight has been connected to an increased risk of type 2 diabetes.

• **Being 45 or older**: Unlike type 1, elderly adults are more prone to acquire type 2 diabetes.

• **Family history**: Having a parent or sibling with type 2 diabetes makes you more likely to have the condition.

- **History of gestational diabetes**: If you've been diagnosed with gestational diabetes during pregnancy or had a baby above nine pounds in weight, you're at increased risk of type 2 diabetes.

- **Race**: Black Americans, Latinx Americans, American Indians, and Alaska Natives are at increased risk of type 2 diabetes.

SYMPTOMS

A tough fact about this disease: Sometimes, there are no signs or symptoms that are so subtle that they're easy to detect. That's why virtually all pregnant women are checked for gestational diabetes, and the U.S. Preventive Services Task Force advises screening for individuals over 40 who have risk factors such as abdominal obesity.

Other times, symptoms are sudden and apparent. Here's what you need to know.

First Signs of Diabetes

Having any of the following indicators does not always imply you have diabetes. Instead, consider these a signal to contact your doctor:

• **Major thirst**: When your blood has too much sugar in it, your body takes water from surrounding tissues to attempt to dilute it. That leaves you dehydrated and thirsty. Some diabetics feel that no matter how much they drink, they can't satiate their thirst.

• **A lot of pee**: When there's too much sugar in the blood, your kidneys try to filter it out. They put it into your urine, making additional pee. In more severe stages of the illness, damaged nerves surrounding the bladder may cause some individuals to feel the desire to pee regularly, even if little or nothing comes out. You also have an increased risk of urinary tract infections (UTIs).

• **Blurry vision**: High blood sugar may lead to a seeping of fluids into your eye, causing the lens to enlarge. That leads to problems concentrating.

• **The munchies**: If you're hungry all the time, even after a decent meal, it might be an indication that your muscles and other tissues aren't receiving the energy—i.e. glucose—they need from the food you're consuming since it's stuck up in your bloodstream. Your muscles inform your brain that they're starving (even if you ate enough), making you hungry again and prolonging the cycle.

• **Increase in infections**: Type 2 diabetes makes it tougher for your immune system to fight off infections, including yeast infections or UTIs. It could also take longer for wounds to heal since additional glucose stops white blood cells from conducting their healing function.

• **Weight loss:** Losing weight without modifying your diet might be an indication of type 1 diabetes. If your body can't acquire the glucose it needs from meals, it will start to break down its own fat, muscles, and other tissues for fuel, resulting in weight loss.

• **Fatigue:** You may feel fatigued and weak because your brain, muscles, and other bodily systems aren't receiving the energy they need to perform correctly. If you're dehydrated, it might make you fatigued, too.

Type 1 Diabetes vs. Type 2 Diabetes Symptoms

When you have type 1 diabetes, your symptoms may start rapidly, taking just a few weeks to build up. In contrast, type 2 diabetes develops considerably more gradually and might take many years. In fact, symptoms may be so minor at first that you don't even know anything is different. That's why it's crucial to have frequent checkups at your doctor—they may be able to spot abnormalities early with blood testing and help prevent type 2 from growing worse.

Diabetes Symptoms in Women

Diabetes may impact you differently depending on your sex. Risks tend to be larger and problems more severe in women. For example, women with diabetes have twice the increased heart disease risk of males. Women also have an increased risk of consequences from diabetes including blindness, renal problems, and even depression.

Women with diabetes also are at high risk of vaginal yeast infections and urinary tract infections. Keeping your blood sugar levels under control may help lessen this danger.

On top of all that, women who menstruate may find their blood sugar levels difficult to anticipate before and after their period because of fluctuating hormones. Those hormone shifts might create challenges in your sex life, too—

talk with your doctor if you're worried about painful sex or low libido.

Finally, diabetes may make it difficult to become pregnant and increase your chance of pregnancy issues. being your diabetes under control before being pregnant is beneficial, along with frequent checks during pregnancy.

Diabetes Symptoms in Men

All that said, guys aren't off the hook when it comes to diabetes. Not only are males more likely to have type 2 diabetes at a lower weight than women, but men are also more likely to have undetected diabetes. So don't put off those routine exams with your doctor, and schedule an appointment if you detect any weird new symptoms.

Your diabetes also triples your chance of acquiring erectile dysfunction (ED).

Thankfully, there are many therapies available to aid with this. Due to nerve damage with diabetes, you also may develop overactive bladder or incontinence, UTIs, or a condition called retrograde ejaculation, which is when semen is expelled into your bladder.

Diabetic Ketoacidosis and Diabetic Coma

In extreme circumstances, your diabetes—in particular, type 1 diabetes—may cause you to develop a condition called diabetic ketoacidosis (DKA). This may happen if your body doesn't obtain enough glucose, so your body begins burning fat to acquire the energy it needs. This process creates compounds called ketones. If ketones build up in the blood, it makes your blood more acidic, and extreme quantities may potentially harm you.

The first warning symptoms of DKA include:

• Having to urinate frequently

• Feeling extremely thirsty or having a dry mouth

• Having high blood glucose levels

• Having large quantities of ketones in the urine

Full-blown DKA leads to the following symptoms:

• Feeling weary all the time

• Dry, flushed skin

• Nausea, vomiting, or stomach pain

• Breath that smells fruity

• Confusion or trouble focusing

• trouble breathing

If you suspect you may have DKA, it's crucial to receive medical care very soon. DKA may progress to diabetic coma, which is when you pass out for a lengthy period, and in the most severe instances, death.

BLOOD SUGAR REGULATION AND STABILIZATION

Maintaining a consistent blood sugar level may be incredibly tough for someone with diabetes. What you consume, your activity level, medications, illness, stress, and even hydration consumption may all play a function in lowering blood glucose rises.

Simple or direct carbohydrate sources promote quick blood sugar increase. Items containing fat are not indicated for treating low blood sugar since they block the release of glucose, delaying therapy and needing more to get the number back to a healthy level. Low blood sugar therapy must be small, accurate, and portable.

It takes time to boost or reduce glucose levels. Overtreatment causes blood glucose to move too far in the other way, generating further difficulties.

The following indicators will alert you to the fact that you have high blood sugar:

• Urination on a regular basis

• Fatigue

• Increased hunger/thirst

• Headaches

• Concentration issues

• Blurry vision

The ranges for high blood sugar vary based on age, how long diabetes has been present, and whether or not other health issues are present. Maintaining blood sugar levels within the range advised by your healthcare practitioner is very crucial.

Methods to Lower Your Blood Sugar Level Immediately

Guiding your blood sugar levels is critical if you have diabetes. Here are some straightforward but practical strategies to reduce your blood glucose levels. However, be sure you've previously taken your insulin or other diabetes medicines. If you miss a dosage, your blood sugar level will plunge.

Drink more water

When you experience a fast blood sugar increase, the first and most crucial thing to do is to check your water level. When your blood sugar levels are high, your body flushes away the extra glucose via the urine.

Consume lots of water instead of juice or fizzy beverages to dilute the blood sugar quality. Furthermore, when you are desiccate, the carbohydrates in your blood become more concentrated.

Walking or Spot Jogging

A simple exercise might help to lessen unexpected blood sugar spikes if you have any indicators of increased glucose levels. To stop the spikes, for example, take a brief walk or gentle jog.

Any aerobic activity can help you regulate your blood glucose levels. Walking for 20 minutes, for example, helps lower blood glucose levels.

Consume Fibre-rich Foods

Certain meals may help maintain blood sugar levels steady throughout the day. High-fiber meals, for example, take longer to digest, which helps to maintain blood sugar levels constant.

Furthermore, studies have shown that fiber-rich foods such as spinach, cereal (such as oats, barley, and others), and avocados may help lower the chances of getting type 2 diabetes.

Cut Down the Simple carbs

Eating too many refined carbs is one of the primary reasons for high blood sugar. These carbs have been processed, and most of the fiber has been removed.

These carbohydrates are promptly digested and absorbed by your body, where they are transformed into sugar. Bread, pasta, rice, and other carb-rich meals should be avoided to prevent blood sugar rises. Choose low-carb veggies, healthy fats, and lean meats instead.

Elevate the Electrolyte Level

You will pee more than usual if your blood sugar level abruptly spikes. It signals that you are losing water and that your electrolyte levels, which include magnesium, potassium, and phosphates, are severely low.

Electrolytes are essential to support correct biological activities, so replenishment is crucial. Bananas, sweet potatoes, and nuts may help you retain your balance.

Get a grip on stress

Another reason for a fast sugar spike in your blood is stress. As a consequence, meditation or yoga will drastically drop blood sugar levels. Breathe during yoga practice to effectively decrease anxiety, quiet the mind, and relax the body.

Fast-acting Insulin

Your doctor suggests fast-acting insulin
to assist moderate the typical blood
sugar spikes that occur when you eat. It
is instantly absorbed by your body and
starts operating to lower high blood
sugar after meals within 15 minutes
after injection.

Fast-acting mealtime insulin, which is
given to patients with type 1 or type 2
diabetes, starts performing quicker than
ordinary human insulin.

Never miss eating breakfast

We have all heard that early meal is the
most important meal of the day. This is
especially true for people who has
diabetes. A high-protein lunch delivers
an edge over a high-carbohydrate
morning. The best early meal includes
protein 39g and resulted in reduced

post-meal glucose spikes than meals with less protein. Furthermore, eating breakfast may enable overweight people with type 2 diabetes to lower their weight.

Add additional resistant starch to your plate

Resistant starch, which is included in certain potatoes and beans, skips the small intestine and ferments in the large intestine, which means it does not boost glucose levels and encourages the development of healthy bacteria in the body. And the impact will persist until your next meal. There are also resistant starches in:

• Unripe bananas and plantains

• Lentils, beans, and peas

• Whole grains, such as oats and barley

Just keep your carb count in mind when introducing resistant starch items into your diet.

Tips to Avoid High Sugar-Level Emergency

The greatest strategy to lower your blood sugar level is to avoid the sugar in the first place. So here are some suggestions to prevent an emergency.

The greatest way to reduce your blood sugar is to prevent the spike in the first place. So here are some ideas to assist you avoid an emergency.

• Avoid sitting or laying down shortly after eating, since this passive action elevates blood sugar levels.

• Don't miss breakfast, the most crucial meal of the day, since it may alter blood glucose levels.

• Getting adequate sleep is vital for preventing blood sugar abnormalities.

• Regular exercise will assist to control blood glucose levels, burning any excess rapidly.

• Consume nutritious meals and nutritional snacks to minimize blood sugar rises.

• Consume foods with a low glycaemic index, such as leafy green vegetables, raw carrots, chickpeas, and lentils, which have minimal effect on glucose levels.

• Keep track of your portion size to prevent overeating and affecting insulin function.

List of foods that boost blood sugar levels

1. White Grains, are a Refined Source of Carbs

2. Sugar-Sweetened Drinks, Which Lack Key Nutrients

3. Fast Food, Which Is an Unexpected Sugar-Bomb & Trans Fats

4. Fruit-flavoured yogurt, Which Can Send Blood Sugar Soaring When Overeaten

5. Starchy Vegetables, Which in high Amounts Can Destabilize Blood Sugar

6. Sweetened morning cereals

7. Flavoured coffee drinks

8. Honey, agave nectar, and maple syrup

9. Packaged snack foods

10. French fries

11. Fruit juice

Knowing which meals to avoid when you have diabetes could be tough at times. However, following a few guidelines may assist.

Your principal objective should be to avoid unhealthy fats, liquid sugars, processed grains, and other foods rich in refined carbs.

Avoiding meals that increase blood sugar levels and cause insulin resistance will help you remain healthy and minimize your chance of future diabetes complications.

DIABETES PREVENTION

Lose additional weight: Losing weight lessens the risk of diabetes. People in one big research lowered their risk of acquiring diabetes by over 60% after decreasing around 7% of their body weight with adjustments in activity and food. Set a weight-loss target depending on your current body weight. Talk to your coach about appropriate short-term objectives and expectations, such as losing 1 to 2 pounds a week.

Be more physically active

There are several advantages to regular physical exercise. Exercise may benefit you:

- Lose weight

- reduce your blood sugar

• Boost your sensitivity to insulin — which helps maintain your blood sugar within a reasonable level

Goals for most individuals to encourage weight reduction and maintain a healthy weight include:

Aerobic workout. Aim for 30 minutes or more of moderate to intense aerobic activity — such as brisk walking, swimming, bicycling, or running — on most days for a total of at least 150 minutes a week.

Resistance exercise. Resistance training — at least 2 to 3 times a week — boosts your strength, balance, and capacity to sustain an active life. Resistance training which includes yoga, weightlifting, and calisthenics.

Limited inactivity. Breaking up extended episodes of inactivity, such as sitting at the computer, may help regulate blood sugar levels. Take a few minutes to stand, stroll around or perform some mild exercise every 30 minutes.

Eat healthful plant foods

Plants give vitamins, minerals, and carbs to your diet. Carbohydrates comprise sugars and carbohydrates – the energy sources for your body — and fiber. Dietary fiber, often known as bulk, is the component of plant foods your body can't process or absorb

Fiber-rich meals improve weight reduction and lessen the risk of diabetes. Eat a range of nutritious, fiber-rich meals, such include:

• Fruits, like tomatoes, peppers, and fruit from trees

• Nonstarchy vegetables, such as leafy greens, and cauliflower

• Legumes, such as beans, chickpeas, and lentils

• Whole grains, these include whole-wheat pasta and bread, whole-grain rice, whole oats, and quinoa

The advantages of fiber include:

• Slowing the absorption of carbohydrates and decreasing blood sugar levels

• Managing other risk factors that impact heart health, such as blood pressure and inflammation

• Helping you eat less since fiber-rich meals are more satisfying and energy-dense

Avoid foods that are "bad carbohydrates" — heavy in sugar with no fiber or nutrients: white bread and pastries, pasta from white flour, fruit juices, and processed foods containing sugar or high-fructose corn syrup.

Eat healthy fats:

Fatty meals are rich in calories and should be taken in moderation. To assist reduce and control weight, your diet should contain a range of foods with unsaturated fats, commonly termed "good fats."

Unsaturated fats — including monounsaturated and polyunsaturated fats — encourage healthy blood cholesterol levels and excellent heart and vascular health. Sources of healthy fats include:

• Olive, sunflower, safflower, and canola oils

• Nuts and seeds, likes almonds, peanuts, flaxseed, and pumpkin seeds

• Fatty fish, which include salmon, mackerel, sardines, tuna, and cod

Saturated fats, the "bad fats," are gotten in dairy products and meats. These should be a tiny portion of your diet. You can reduce saturated fats by eating low-fat dairy products and lean chicken and pork.

Skip fad diets and choose better choices:

Many trendy diets — such as the glycemic index, paleo, or keto diets — may help you lose weight. There is no data, however, on the long-term advantages of these diets or their efficacy in avoiding diabetes.

Your eating objective should be to reduce weight and then maintain a healthy weight going forward. Healthy food selections, then, need to incorporate a technique that you can keep as a lifetime habit. Making healthy selections that reflect some of your personal tastes in food and customs may be helpful for you over time.

One easy method to help you make excellent food choices and consume proper quantities and sizes is to split up your plate. These three divisions on your plate encourage healthy eating:

• One-half: fruit and nonstarchy vegetables

• One-quarter: whole grains

• One-quarter: protein-rich foods, such as legumes, seafood, or lean meats

• People younger than 45 who are overweight and have risk factors associated with diabetes

• Women who have had gestational diabetes

• People who have been confirmed with prediabetes

• Children who are overweight and who have a family background of type 2 diabetes or other risk factors

DIABETES MANAGEMENT

How lifestyle, and everyday routine affect blood sugar

Diabetes control demands awareness. Know what causes your blood sugar level to increase and decrease — and how to handle these day-to-day issues.

Keeping your blood sugar levels within the range prescribed by your doctor might be tough. That's because numerous factors make your blood sugar levels vary, often suddenly. Following are some things that might alter your blood sugar levels.

Food

Healthy nutrition is a cornerstone of healthy life — with or without diabetes. But if you have diabetes, you need to know how meals impact your blood sugar levels. It's not just the sort of food you consume, but also how much you eat and the combinations of food types you eat.

What to do:

Learn about carbohydrate counting and portion proportions. A fundamental to many diabetes control strategies is learning how to measure carbs. Carbohydrates frequently have the most influence on your blood sugar levels. For persons using mealtime insulin, it's crucial to know the quantity of carbs in your diet, so you receive the right insulin dosage.

Learn what portion size is suitable for each meal type. Simplify your meal planning by jotting down servings for things you consume regularly. Use measuring cups or a scale to ensure adequate portion size and an exact carbohydrate count.

Make every meal properly balanced. As much as possible, prepare every meal to incorporate a decent balance of carbs, fruits and vegetables, proteins, and fats. Pay attention to the sorts of carbs you pick.

Some carbs, such as fruits, vegetables, and whole grains, are healthier for you than others. These meals are low in carbs and feature fiber that helps keep your blood sugar levels more consistent. Talk to your doctor, nurse, or nutritionist about the optimal meal choices and the proper mix of food kinds.

Coordinate your meals and prescriptions. Too few meals in proportion to your diabetes treatments — particularly insulin — may result in dangerously low blood sugar (hypoglycemia). Too much eating may cause your blood sugar level to soar too high (hyperglycemia).

Avoid sugar-sweetened drinks. Sugar-sweetened drinks tend to be heavy in calories and provide little nutrients. And since they cause blood sugar to increase fast, it's better to avoid certain sorts of beverages if you have diabetes.

Exercise

Physical exercise is another key aspect of your diabetes control regimen. When you work out, your muscles need sugar (glucose) for energy. Regular physical exercise also helps your body handle insulin more effectively.

These elements work together to lower your blood sugar level. The more rigorous your exercise, the longer the impact lasts. But even modest tasks — such as cleaning, gardening, or standing for long periods — could help increase your blood sugar.

What to do:

Talk to your doctor about an activity regimen. Ask your doctor about what form of exercise is acceptable for you. In general, most individuals should obtain at least 150 minutes a week of moderate aerobic exercise. Aim for roughly 30 minutes of moderate aerobic exercise a day on most days of the week.

If you have not been active for a long time, your doctor may want your full body health check before giving you advise. He or she may propose the correct combination of aerobic and muscle-strengthening activities.

Keep an exercise regimen. Talk to your doctor about the optimum time of day for you to exercise so that your workout program is coordinated with your food and prescription routines.

Know your numbers. Talk to your doctor about what blood sugar levels are acceptable for you before you begin activity.

Check your blood sugar level. Check your blood sugar level before, during, and after exercise, particularly if you use insulin or drugs that reduce blood sugar. Exercise may drop your blood sugar levels even up to a day later, particularly if the activity is new to you, or if you're exercising at a higher severe level. Be alert of warning indications of low blood sugar, such as feeling shaky, weak, weary, hungry, lightheaded, irritated, nervous, or confused.

If you use insulin and your blood sugar level is below 90 milligrams per deciliter or 5.0 millimoles per liter, ingest a short snack before you start exercising to avoid a low blood sugar level.

Stay hydrated. Drink lots of water or other fluids when exercising since dehydration might impact blood sugar levels.

Be prepared. Always bring a little snack or glucose tablets with you while exercising in case your blood sugar level gets too low. Wear a medical identification bracelet.

Adjust your diabetes treatment regimen as required. If you use insulin, you may need to lower your insulin dosage before exercising and check your blood sugar carefully for many hours after vigorous exercise since occasionally delayed hypoglycemia may develop. Your doctor can advise you on suitable modifications to your medication. You may also need to change therapy if you've upped your workout program.

Medication

Insulin and other diabetic drugs are meant to reduce your blood sugar levels when diet and exercise alone aren't adequate for treating diabetes. But the success of these treatments relies on the time and quantity of the dosage. Medications you take for diseases other than diabetes also might alter your blood sugar levels.

What to do:

Store insulin appropriately. Insulin that's incorrectly kept or beyond its expiry date may not be effective. Insulin is extremely sensitive to fluctuations in temperature.

Report issues to your doctor. If your diabetic drugs cause your blood sugar level to dip too low or if it's continuously too high, the dose or time may need to be modified.

Be careful with new drugs. whether you're contemplating an over-the-counter medicine or your doctor prescribes a new treatment to address another problem — such as high blood pressure or high cholesterol — ask your doctor or pharmacist whether the medication may influence your blood sugar levels.

Sometimes an alternative drug may be prescribed. Always check with your doctor before taking any new over-the-counter medicine, so you know how it may affect your blood sugar level.

Illness

When you're unwell, your body creates stress-related chemicals that help your body fight the sickness, but they also may elevate your blood sugar level. Changes in your appetite and daily activity also may affect diabetes control.

What to do:

Plan ahead. Work with your healthcare team to build a sick-day strategy. Include instructions on what drugs to take, how frequently to monitor your blood sugar and urine ketone levels, how to alter your medication doses, and when to contact your doctor.

Continue to take your diabetic treatment. However, if you're unable to eat due to nausea or vomiting, consult your doctor. In rare situations, you may need to temporarily decrease or withhold short-acting insulin or diabetic treatment because of a risk of hypoglycemia. However, do not quit your long-acting insulin. During times of sickness, it is vital to test your blood glucose often, and your doctor may urge you also to check your urine for the presence of ketones.

Stick to your diabetic eating plan. If you can, eating as normal will help you regulate your blood sugar levels. Keep a supply of items that are soft on your stomach, such as gelatin, crackers, soups, and applesauce.

Drink plenty of water or other fluids that don't add calories, which include tea, to ensure you keep hydrated.

Alcohol

The liver generally releases stored sugar to counteract falling blood sugar levels. But if your liver is metabolizing alcohol, your blood sugar level may not receive the boost it needed from your liver. Alcohol can result in low blood sugar right after you consume it and for as long as 24 hours afterwards.

What to do:

Get your doctor's OK to consume alcohol. Alcohol may increase diabetic problems, such as nerve damage and eye discomfort. But if your diabetes is under manage and your doctor accept, an infrequent alcoholic drink is OK.

Moderate alcohol intake is defined as no more than one drink (One drink equals a 12-ounce beer, 5 ounces of wine, or 1.5 ounces of distilled liquor) a day for ladies of any age and guys over 65 years old and two drinks a day for males under 65.

Don't consume alcoholic drinks on an empty stomach. If you take insulin or other diabetic drugs, be sure to eat before you drink, or drink with a meal to prevent low blood sugar.

Choose your beverages carefully. Light beer and dry wines contain fewer calories and carbs than other alcoholic beverages.

Tally your calories. Remember to add the calories from any alcohol you consume to your daily calorie total. Ask your doctor how to integrate calories from alcoholic beverages into your diet plan.

Check your blood sugar level before night. Because alcohol may drop blood sugar levels confirm your blood sugar level before you go to sleep long after you've had your last drink. If your blood sugar isn't between 100 and 140 mg/dL (5.6 and 7.8 mmol/L), consume a snack before night to offset a decline in your blood sugar level.

Menstruation and menopause

Changes in hormone levels the week before and during menstruation could result in large changes in blood sugar levels.

What to do:

Look for trends. Keep attentive note of your blood sugar levels from month

to month. You may be able to foresee
swings connected to your menstrual
cycle.

**Adjust your diabetes treatment
regimen as appropriate**. Your doctor
may prescribe modifications in your
dietary plan, exercise level, or diabetic
medicines to make up for blood sugar
variance.

Check blood sugar more routinely.
whether you're probably nearing
menopause or experiencing menopause,
chat to your doctor about whether you
need to check your blood sugar level
more regularly. Signs of menopause
may be misinterpreted with symptoms
of low blood sugar, therefore wherever
practicable, test your blood sugar before
treating a suspected low to confirm the
low blood

Most types of birth control may be used by women with diabetes without a problem. However, oral contraceptives may boost blood sugar levels in certain women.

Stress

If you're stressed, the chemicals your body creates in reaction to persistent stress may induce a jump in your blood sugar level. Additionally, it may be tough to appropriately follow your usual diabetes treatment plan if you're under a lot of additional strain.

What to do:

Look for trends. record your stress level on a scale of 1 to 10 each time you report your blood sugar level. A pattern may soon emerge.

Take charge. Once you realize how stress influences your blood sugar level, fight back. Learn calming techniques, prioritize your chores, and impose limitations. Whenever possible, avoid usual tensions. Exercise may generally aid minimize tension and lower your blood sugar level.

Get assistance. Learn new ways for managing stress. You may discover that chatting with a psychologist or clinical social worker may help you recognize stress, manage stressful conditions, or learn new coping skills.

The more you know about things that impact your blood sugar level, the more you can forecast variations – and prepare correctly. If you're encountering difficulty managing your blood sugar level in your ideal range, contact your diabetic healthcare team for support.

TREATMENT

How Do Doctors Diagnose Diabetes?

Getting diagnosed with diabetes includes blood tests and maybe extra testing to find out which type you have. Correct diagnosis is vital as therapy changes dependent on the type.

What to Expect at the Doctor's Office

It's fair to be nervous as you travel to your doctor's visit to review a possible diagnosis of diabetes. Knowing what you may anticipate throughout your session will help lessen the anxiousness. Your doctor will likely undertake a physical exam and ask you questions about your symptoms and family history. Typically, the initial line of action to screen for diabetes is to take a blood test.

Blood Tests for Diabetes

The first step in acquiring a diabetes diagnosis is a blood test. There are various conceivable types.

A1C (or Glycated Hemoglobin) Test

This frequent test evaluates what proportion of your red blood cells have been coated with glucose during the preceding two to three months. The greater your blood sugar, the higher your score. An A1C value below 5.7 is considered normal; 5.7 to 6.4 is prediabetic; 6.5 or higher implies diabetes.

Fasting Blood Sugar Test

Blood will be drawn first thing in the morning before your meal or drink anything other than water. A test under 100 milligrams per deciliter is normal; 100 to 125 mg/dL is prediabetic; 126 mg/dL or higher suggests diabetes. Your doctor will likely want to run the test twice before diagnosing you.

Glucose Tolerance Test

After having your blood taken on an empty stomach, you'll sip a glucose drink, then have blood drawn again after one or two hours. If your blood sugar is under 140 mg/dL two hours after downing the sugar drink, that's acceptable; 140 to 199 is prediabetic; 200 md/dL or higher signals diabetes.

Random Blood Sugar Test

Blood is taken at any time of day, whether you've eaten lately or not. A result of 200 mg/dL implies you may have diabetes.

Antibody Test

To assist distinguish between type 1 and type 2 diabetes, your doctor may also sample blood for an "autoantibody" test, to examine whether your immune system is attacking your pancreas. People with type 1 frequently test positive for multiple particular autoantibodies, but those with type 2 (or the uncommon monogenic diabetes) won't.

Urine Test for Diabetes

If your doctor believes that you have type 1 diabetes, she may want to test your urine for ketones, molecules your body makes as it breaks down fat for energy.

The test may be done at home or at a lab or doctor's office by peeing into a specimen cup. Extremely high amounts of ketones are an indication of ketoacidosis, a potentially deadly complication of diabetes that needs immediate care.

Treatment

Whatever your course of treatment, most likely you'll start by measuring your glucose every day, or possibly many times each day, in order to make judgments about insulin doses, diet, and exercise. This is an entire lifestyle so we'll break it down in depth after we speak about other therapies. Beyond self-monitoring, here are a few sorts of therapies your doctor will examine, depending on your diabetes type:

Type 1 Diabetes Treatments

The main therapy for type 1 diabetes is insulin. Here's everything you need to know.

Insulin

people with type 1 diabetes requires insulin daily. There are a handful of various ways insulin may be given to the body:

• **Injection**: To give yourself an injection, the most frequent form of getting insulin, the medicine, you will need a syringe or "pen." This will be inserted in your abdomen, upper arm, thigh, or butt.

• **Insulin pump**: People who require numerous injections per day or are at high risk of ketoacidosis may choose an insulin pump, which automatically administers insulin throughout the day via a small catheter that's worn on your body.

• **Insulin inhaler**: Some individuals with type 1 or 2 diabetes may also use inhaled insulin, a powder you breathe into your lungs using an inhaler.

The Dangers of Too Much Insulin

Accidentally taking too much insulin is dangerous—it may cause your blood sugar to fall and lead to hypoglycemia. This may happen if you mistakenly inject the incorrect dosage at the wrong time, or inject your insulin but then miss your usual meal thereafter. If you've overdosed on insulin, it's crucial to seek medical attention straight soon. In the most extreme circumstances, an insulin overdose may lead to convulsions or coma.

Treatment for Type 2 Diabetes

How you go about controlling your disease will rely on several aspects, including your blood sugar patterns, medical history, lifestyle, commitments, economics, and personal preferences. Your doctor will chat with you about several strategies to treat the condition, including:

Eating Smart

While there's no official diet for diabetes, it should go without saying that sugary, fatty meals are not what your body needs when it's already suffering from high blood sugar.

Research reveals that plant-based diets, Mediterranean diets (high in vegetables and fish), and low-carbohydrate diets may all decrease blood sugar and minimize the likelihood of getting type 2 diabetes or improve symptoms if you already have it.

doubtful how to start one of these programs? A registered dietitian or certified diabetes educator can help you plan meals based on these concepts and find out how to integrate healthy eating into your budget and lifestyle.

Exercising

No one's asking you to summit Everest here, but if you want to overcome this illness, you've got to move! Exercise boosts your blood sugar levels by making your cells more receptive to insulin—even a regular stroll around the block may assist.

Besides, national standards call for a minimum of 150 minutes weekly of moderate exercise (that's 30 minutes a day, five days a week), so even if you didn't have type 2, you still requires to get up and move.

Taking Oral Medications

If you have type 2 diabetes, there's a possibility you will be able to regulate your blood sugar with exercise and what you eat. But you may require medicine, too.

There are a variety of different treatments that might help decrease blood sugar—your doctor could suggest one, or a combination of medications, depending on your unique condition.

Checking Blood Glucose Some persons with type 2 diabetes may need to check their blood glucose infrequently, others need to do it numerous times a day.

Most individuals use a home glucose meter to achieve this. To use it, you puncture a fingertip with a specialized lancet "pen" and then drop the blood onto a test strip in the meter. For certain persons who have to check readings regularly, it makes more sense to use a continuous glucose monitor (CGM). A CGM is a small sensor put under the skin of your belly, arms, or thighs that examines glucose levels in bodily fluids periodically and will notify you if levels go too low.

Getting Blood Tests

People with type 2 diabetes should undergo an A1C (or glycated hemoglobin) test two to four times each year. If levels go higher, your doctor may opt to alter your medicines or advise you to place more focus on your diet and activity objectives.

Living With Type 2 Diabetes

Because of the links between type 2 diabetes, BMI, and physical activity, there's sometimes a false notion that persons with the illness have caused their condition themselves.

To be clear, eating too much takeout or sitting on the sofa does not cause type 2 diabetes. A bad diet and lack of exercise certainly raise your risk, but there are other variables at play. Two individuals may be overweight, have a strong family history, sedentary lifestyle, and consume fast food—and one will acquire type 2, while the other won't. Type 2 diabetes is a complicated condition with various causes and (fortunately) remedies.

The truly good news is that many of those answers are things you can do beginning right now. Along with medicine, you may considerably enhance your chances of lowering type 2 symptoms and living a full and happy life by adopting a Mediterranean or plant-based diet, limiting your intake of high-sugar foods, and squeezing in 30 minutes of moderate exercise, five days a week. No one is claiming it's easy, but neither is life with type 2 diabetes. Start making adjustments immediately. You've got this.